THE TREATMENT OF CATS
BY HOMOEOPATHY

THE TREATMENT OF CATS BY HOMOEOPATHY

by

K. SHEPPARD

illustrated by

Stephen Brown

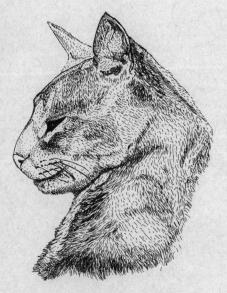

HEALTH SCIENCE PRESS

The C. W. Daniel Company Limited,
1 Church Path,
Saffron Walden,
Essex CB10 1JP.

First published as *The Homoeopathic
Treatment of Cats* in 1960
First Paperback Edition December 1974
Illustrated edition October 1979

ISBN 0 85032 120 4

*Made and Printed in Great Britain by
Weatherby Woolnough, Wellingborough
Northants, England, NN8 4BX*

INTRODUCTION

Hippocrates stated "Disease is produced by its similar, and by the similars which are administered the patient returns from disease to good health . . . fever is produced by what it suppresses, and suppressed by what it produces."

Paracelsus: "The names of diseases do not serve to indicate remedies, it is the similar which has to be compared with its similar . . . and that comparison serves to reveal the secrets of healing."

This law was proved once again true by Hahnemann well over 100 years ago. He experimented upon himself, while in good health, with Peruvian Bark, and found that it produced a fever similar to Malaria. He then repeated this experiment on other healthy people and obtained the same results. He continued these experiments, with hundreds of other substances, on other healthy subjects. The result was always the same; medicines administered in strong doses to the healthy produced symptoms similar to those which were made to disappear in the sick man. From this, the Law of Similars was re-established, and Homoeopathy, as it is known today, was established.

There is a very common belief among those who know nothing about it that Homoeopathy consists of simply giving medicines in very small doses. In fact, Homoeopathy differs radically from Allopathic medicine not only in the size of the dose, but in the principle on which the remedies are selected. This principle is that what produces the symptoms if administered in large doses, will cure if given in small ones. Hahnemann by his own experience observed that the smaller the dose, the greater the effect.

Why the efficacy of the infinitesimal dose should be doubted seems odd, since orthodox medicine so readily admits the havoc wrought by the "invisible and infiltrable virus."

That the Law of Similars is gaining ground is proved by the present trend of inoculations with disease products.

Homoeopathy proves its remedies on healthy people. It does not use animals for experiments. The medicines used by Hahnemann over 100 years ago are still used, with the same results.

The ideal is first to find the totality of the symptoms and then to find the medicine to cover them. The times of amelioration or aggravation are of enormous help if these can be observed in an animal—which they often can with careful observation while nursing a sick cat.

One must individualise and remember that it is the sick cat that one is trying to cure, not a named disease, which may present as many different symptoms as there are cats affected.

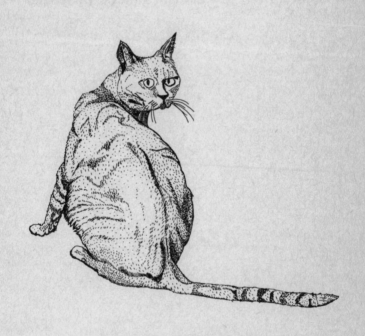

ABSCESS

Cats are rather prone to abscesses. They often get them on the face and this may be due—especially in old cats—to a bad tooth, which should be attended to and, if necessary, extracted by a veterinary surgeon (see Teeth), or on the throat or neck or anywhere on the body. They also develop septic conditions as the result of scratches and fights.

In some cases these conditions may be accompanied by high temperature, and the cat is obviously in pain and very ill.

TREATMENT: Bathe with warm *Calendula Lotion* (one teaspoonful of Calendula Ø to half a cup of hot water), every 3 hours. Give *Tarentula Cubensis 30*, internally at hourly intervals, this eases the pain in an astonishing manner and brings the abscess to a head speedily, and will sometimes abort it.

When the abscess has opened and is discharging, apply locally a compress of *Calendula Lotion* (as above) and keep it in place with a bandage; change the lint frequently. When the bulk of the discharge has come away, use *Calendula Ointment* instead of the lotion.

If *Tarentula Cubensis* is not available, *Belladonna 6* at two hourly intervals will relieve the pain and bring the abscess to a head, when it begins to discharge, give *Hepar Sulph 6* every two or three hours and apply *Hepar Sulph* ointment to clear away the rest of the discharge.

ANAEMIA

Cats often show signs of anaemia after acute illness or loss of blood. The symptoms are: Gums paler than usual, in cats with pink noses the nose is almost white, the cat is listless.

TREATMENT: If it develops after acute illness give *Calcium Phos 3x* or *Natrum Mur 6x*, three times a day, this will improve the condition. In addition give plenty of nourishing food and see that the cat gets fresh air. If the anaemia is the result of loss of blood, give *China 3* every four hours.

ASTHMA

Old cats sometimes suffer from asthma; the symptoms are cough and laboured or spasmodic breathing.

TREATMENT: If worse at night, worse in a warm room or by changes of temperature, either hot or cold, or worse moving, give *Sulphur 30*, one dose only, repeat when necessary.

If the condition is worse by any kind of exertion, the cat hugs the fire and is better by warmth, yet seeks cold water to drink, give *Arsenicum Album 30*, one dose only will relieve the symptoms.

Should the cat cough and vomit saliva like beaten white of egg, *Ipecacuanha 3* every half hour will alleviate, or *Bryonia 6* every two hours if the animal is better lying still and is decidedly thirsty.

Spongia 1x every two hours is called for when there is panting, difficult respiration with suffocative cough. DO NOT repeat the dose while the improvement is maintained.

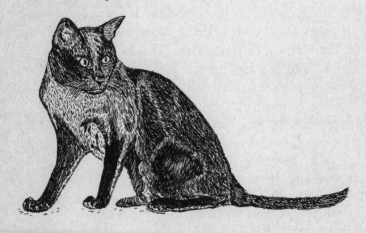

BLADDER-INFLAMMATION (Cystitis)

Symptoms: This is often the result of a chill and if taken in time *Rhus Toxicodendron* 6 at two hourly intervals may cut it short but, as a rule, it is not noticed until it has gone too far. Then the cat is always demanding to be let out, it strains and passes only a few drops of urine.

Give *Apis 3x* every two hours when there is frequent and involuntary urination which is scanty and high coloured.

Cantharis 3 every two hours where there is intolerable urging and constant desire to urinate. The urine might be bloody and there is great pain.

Terebinthina 3 at half-hourly intervals. This is particularly indicated where there is bloody urine, and in cases of inflamed kidneys following any acute disease such at cat influenza.

Neutered males sometimes suffer from gravel, this blocks the urinary passage causing the cat the strain to pass urine. The distended bladder can be felt like a hard ball at the lower back of the abdomen, it feels warm and is sensitive to touch. It is obvious that the animal is suffering mentally and physically and it loses condition very quickly. In these cases *Thlaspi Bursa* Ø, two or three drops every half hour will often render the use of the catheter unnecessary.

BRONCHITIS

This is a fairly common trouble in cats during wet or cold weather. It is generally accompanied by a rise in temperature, a sore throat, cough, wheezy breathing and dribbling from the mouth. The animal is generally too distressed to take food.

TREATMENT: Aconite 30, a dose every four hours will often cut short an attack if it is caused by a sudden sharp, cold spell of weather. If there is no improvement within 12 hours this is not the remedy.

Give *Rhus Tox 6* every two hours if the attack is due to damp, or *Bryonia 6* every two hours if the cough is dry and the cat worse by movement or is thirsty. The cat should be kept in an even temperature, free from draughts, with an open window.

BURNS AND SCALDS

A cat may be scalded or burned by jumping into unsuitable places owing to its inherent restless curiosity, and it is not only burnt but badly shocked by any such accident.

TREATMENT: If the burn or scald is not a severe one, quickly apply a large piece of warmed cotton wool to the burned area and give, internally, *Urtica Urens 30* and this can be repeated in 2 to 4 hours or when the animal shows signs of a return of the pain.

Should the burn or scald be more than superficial, apply *Urtica Urens Ø* locally (one teaspoonful to a pint of water, or 20 drops to a large cup of water), soak a pad of lint or gauze in this, cover with cotton wool and bandage. Remove the cotton wool when the dressing feels dry and re-soak the lint or gauze (without removing it) with a few drops of the lotion. *Urtica Urens* relieves the pain very quickly.

CANKER OF THE EAR

Cats get two forms of Canker. The more common form is really eczematous and it is due to overheating of the system in general. The other form is due to a parasite.

A cat with either form of Canker shakes its head and scratches BEHIND the ear, often causing a bare patch; this sore heals quickly when the ear is attended to and the irritation allayed. The ear itself becomes hot and there is an accumulation of a dark wax discharge in the ear.

TREATMENT: Clean out the ear thoroughly with a piece of cotton wool on small tweezers or a match stick; it is, of course, necessary to use fresh cotton wool each time it is withdrawn. Then insert a little *Calendula Ointment.* Continue daily until the ears are cured.

The same treatment is suitable for the parasitical form of canker which is, however, *very contagious.* Here the discharge is dryer and greyer in colour, and the mites can be seen moving about quite easily. This form in particular will sometimes cause a kind of paralysis in the cat, the cat carries its head to one side, it moves as if intoxicated and after a few steps will fall on its side.

In both cases give internally a dose of *Sulphur 200*, which may be repeated in a week if the condition is not by then quite cleared.

Sometimes there is a very offensive acrid persistent discharge from the ear, then *Tellurium 30* is the remedy *par excellence*, given one dose every two or three days over a long period. A cat requiring *Tellurium* usually has some skin symptoms as well as ear trouble and it is particularly difficult to handle as it is very sensitive and afraid of being touched.

CATARRH (Chronic)

This is sometimes the result of a simple cold or an attack of feline influenza, a cat gets a very obstinate form of catarrh; it discharges constantly from its nose, sneezes and blows out mattery discharge. This condition, occasionally, if it is not very bad may clear up spontaneously, but if it does not, treatment must be given.

TREATMENT: (1) if the cat is timid and very amiable and is always *worse in a warm room*, one dose of *Pulsatilla 30* every two or three days for a couple of weeks or longer will often clear the catarrh. (2) If the cat is *worse from dry cold winds, better for warmth,* a dose of *Hepar Sulphuris 30* every two or three days, again for some weeks, should help to cure. (3) If the first two remedies do not cure *Silicea 30* will generally do so, if given in the same way. The *Silicea* patient lacks vital heat, suffers from the cold and hugs the fire. (4)

There are some cases with stoppage of the nose, troublesome eyes, an acrid discharge, and the edges of the lids are red; *Psorinum 200*, one dose, will often clear up all these symptoms.

Rhino-Antipeol put up the nostrils two or three times a day is very helpful. This is supplied by The Medico-Biological Laboratories Ltd., Cargreen Road, South Norwood, London, S.E.25. (6) In cases where the cat has been overdosed without good results, *Teucrium Marum 6*, three times a day, may cure.

CHOKING

Cats sometimes become choked by fish or other small bones. Sometimes one becomes lodged across the palate, the cat claws at its mouth and shows signs of distress so that it is generally quickly noticeable.

Upon opening the mouth one can usually see the bone and remove it with forceps or the end of a fork or spoon quite easily.

Should a small bone or needle or any such obstruction get into the throat this is a matter for veterinary assistance, as an anæsthetic may be needed to remove it.

A few doses of *Arnica Montana 6* will cure any abrasions to the skin and help to allay the shock to the system after removal of the object.

COLDS

Cats are very subject to colds which are contagious. If there is more than one cat it is advisable to isolate the one with the cold at once.

The symptoms are sneezing and watering eyes and nose. With a simple cold there is little or no temperature but the cat should be kept indoors otherwise it might develop bronchitis or pneumonia.

Unless checked in the early stages, the discharge turns to a thick mucus and the cat may develop chronic catarrh, which is not easy to cure.

Colds are usually caused by sudden changes in the weather. The absence of temperature helps to distinguish a simple cold from cat influenza. The cat with a simple cold, though uncomfortable, does not appear to be very ill, nor does it, as a rule, lose its appetite.

TREATMENT: Aconite 30, a dose every four hours for 3 doses in all if the cold follows a sudden cold spell. If there is no improvement and the watery symptoms are marked, try *Kali Iod 1x* every two hours in alternation with *Belladonna 1x.*

Should the trouble follow a cold, damp spell

and the cat sneezes a lot, give *Gelsemium 6* three times a day. Gelsemium suits cats particularly well.

If the discharge has become thick, yellow-green, give *Merc Sol 6* three times a day.

CONSTIPATION

Cats leading a natural life seldom suffer from constipation, but occasionally this occurs. If this is allowed to continue it may lead to a temporary paralysis of the hind legs.

Very often milk alone will be all that is needed as, with many cats, its acts as an aperient. If, however, this should not suffice, give *Nux Vomica 6* every two hours or, for large, hard, dry stools, *Bryonia Alb 6* at two hourly intervals. If the motions are in small, hard pieces give Opium 3 every six hours.

Olive oil mixed in the food, if the cat does not object, or given by mouth in teaspoon doses once or twice a day will often alleviate the condition or help to pass a hairball which could cause an obstruction.

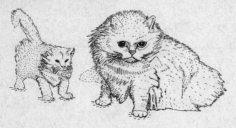

COUGHS

Cats easily get coughs, no doubt owing to their habit of sitting in the warmest places and then going out to sit on a wall gazing into space. As a rule they are not ill with a cough, though it is wise to keep them in for fear it should lead to something more serious.

TREATMENT: *Bryonia* 6 every two hours for a few doses will generally clear up a dry cough or, if it is spasmodic, *Arsenicum Alb* 6 three times a day.

Some cats cough because they have worms and in these cases *Cina 3* at four hourly intervals is indicated.

DIARRHOEA

This is quite a common complaint in cats. It may be due to simple indigestion or, in kittens, worms or teething can cause the upset.

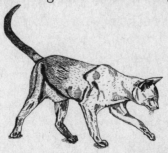

It also occurs in the more serious diseases to which cats are prone so that it should never be overlooked.

Old cats not uncommonly suffer from chronic diarrhœa, which may be due to various causes.

TREATMENT: For very amiable cats with "no two stools alike", *Pulsatilla 6* works like a charm, a dose every two hours.

Where stools are very offensive, acrid, small, liquid and sometimes bloody, and the cat appears ill, restless and depressed, seeks the warmth, give *Arsenicum Alb 3* every four hours *but do not continue this remedy if there is no improvement within 48 hours.*

If the stools are larger and blood-streaked, and the depression not so marked, give *Mercurius Corrosivus 6* at four hourly intervals.

When the stools are grey or white coloured, give *Phosphorus 3x* every two hours.

Where there are solid hard lumps in watery diarrhœa, give *Antimonium Crudum 6* at two hourly intervals.

If the stools are watery yellow, give *Podophyllum 6* every two hours.

Green, chopped white and yellow mucus indicate the need for *Chamomilla 6* two to four hourly.

If the attack occurs in damp, cold weather, give *Dulcamara 6* every two or three hours.

DISTEMPER or INFLUENZA

This is a very infectious disease. It takes various forms and is always accompanied by a sharp rise in temperature which helps to distinguish the catarrhal form from the common cold.

It is now assumed that infectious enteritis is a different complaint from ordinary cat influenza; nevertheless, it is not at all uncommon for some kittens to show catarrhal symptoms and others, at the same time, to be affected with the symptoms of infectious enteritis. However, for the latter see under that heading.

In one form of cat distemper, the initial infection is quite often missed as there are no marked symptoms of any kind except lassitude, rapid wasting and a high temperature of about 105°. The cat just lies about and refuses to move, and prefers to be alone. All the bodily functions appear to be at a standstill and within a few days the cat will become very weak.

TREATMENT: Feed twice a day with raw meat, cut up small and pushed down the throat (about 1 or 2 ozs for an adult cat). For kittens, shredded raw meat is better and I have found that pressing this in at the side of the mouth with a wooden skewer will often induce them to take it, even if they are too weak, or idle, to assist, though at first they invariably give one no assistance.

There are very few symptoms in this form beyond the marked inactivity and disinclination to be kept warm.

Give *Sulphur 30* morning and evening for as long as the temperature keeps up.

The catarrhal form begins in very much the same way as a common cold, but there is a rise of temperature of several degrees, the cat refuses its foods, appears dull and shivery, and sneezes with watery discharge from the nose, and the eyes are watery. The treatment for these conditions is *Gelsemium 30* at four hourly intervals; a cat requiring this remedy is not thirsty and the attack often follows damp, cold weather. Should the symptoms appear after exposure to dry cold weather and be noticed early, *Aconite 30* at four hourly intervals might cut it short but do not continue with this remedy if there is no improvement within 24 hours. As the cat is not a fussy animal and prefers to retire when it is sick, this first stage is often missed and, in the next stage the eyes get more inflamed and they are very sensitive to light and in these circumstances *Belladonna 30* at four hourly intervals, is the indicated remedy.

Should this stage be missed and the cat shows

signs of difficult breathing, temperature remains high and the animal hates to move, it has a dry cough, is thirsty and may drink cold water while still declining food, give *Bryonia 3* in alternation with *Phosphorus 3* at two-hourly intervals but as improvement takes place lengthen the period between doses.

When the cat is very prostrated yet restless, thirsty for small sips of cold water and has very offensive diarrhœa, with small dark or dysenteric motions and a dry, red tongue, all discharges are very offensive then *Arsenicum Alb 30* every four hours for three doses only, may help the animal to recover. The time signal for *Arsenicum Alb* is often helpful, it is "worse after midnight or after noon until 2 p.m."

Similarly the indication for *Phosphorus* is "worse at twilight" (this very marked symptom once guided me to the remedy and cure of a very sick cat).

There is another form of distemper very similar to the last, but the breath is fetid and the tongue has a burned, dry and brown appearance with the edges red and shining, the animal is extremely prostrated with putrid phenomena.

The treatment for this state is *Baptisia 3x* every hour.

If the cat is as ill as in the last two cases it is, of course, quite unable to assimilate solid food. Give Brands' Essence, Slippery Elm food, Honey water or Glucose and water in very small quantities of a teaspoonful or desertspoonful every two to four hours (according to the size of the cat), given at the side of the mouth with a hypodermic syringe from which the needle has been removed. This upsets the cat very little and all feeding, cleaning up and dosing can be done at the same time. Sometimes a teaspoonful of orange juice seems to be acceptable.

I have saved very young kittens, which have very little resistance to this infection, and the kittens were moribund, with one dose of *Pyrogen 30*. This remedy is amazing, for the kittens were all but dead, quite cold, with temperature very sub-normal, and obstinate constipation. The guiding symptoms here are that the pulse is out of proportion to the temperature and the animal smells like death.

With the catarrhal form the cat often gets a very sore throat and dribbles saliva and it is exceedingly sorry for itself. This form is quite common; the cat is very ill and being essentially a cleanly animal, it hates the mess it is in. The throat is dark red or bluish; there is probably difficult breathing, a dry cough; it is generally worse at night, better for warmth and rest. *Phytolacca 30* every four hours will soon relieve most of the symptoms.

For the treatment of eye and chronic catarrh see under those headings.

ECZEMA

This disease is fairly common in cats. It is not contagious. It is often a constitutional disease and very obstinate, at other times it may be caused by unsuitable diet or worms, or too close confinement. The symptoms vary.

There are two kinds of eczema: the dry variety consists of a dry skin and the coat looks dull and there is a lot of scurf in the hair, the cat's skin is irritated, it feels hot and the animal scratches a lot.

This type of eczema may sometimes be cured by a complete change of diet. If the cat has been fed mainly on fish, a change to meat may clear it up. In the form just described *Natrum Muriaticum 6x* morning and evening will often be of help, particularly if it shows signs of anaemia. *Arsenicum Alb 3* morning and evening may help or a single dose of *Arsenicum Alb 30* or *200* and not repeated for a week may give the desired effect, especially if the skin is scaly and it seems painful after scratching. The first remedy mentioned (*Natrum Muriaticum*) might be better where there is a dirty looking skin, and it may be a little withered.

The moist variety, where the skin is red and irritated, the cat licks and makes sore, sticky places, the animal feels hot to the touch, dislikes warmth and looks unthrifty, give *Sulphur 6* morning and evening until the condition shows improvement and then, when most of the symptoms have cleared up give one single dose of *Sulphur 200* which should clear up the complaint. *Calendula ointment* applied to the sore patches relieves the irritation, or diluted *T.C.P.* is very healing and helps the hair to grow on bald patches.

If the eczema is due to worms, treat for that complaint.

EYES

Cats are not particularly prone to eye troubles. They may, however, get them injured in fights and they frequently get inflamed with catarrhal influenza. They can, of course, also get inflammation through dust or sawdust, or from exposure to cold winds or draughts.

In cases of injury bathe with *Calendula lotion* just warm (five drops of Calendula Ø to a wineglass of water), this is very soothing and heals quickly. It should be used three times a day. Internally, give a dose of *Arnica 6* three times a day.

In catarrhal influenza I have found *Influ-*

enzinum 30, every second or third day, to be more helpful than anything else where the eyes are very mattery and sore, and bathe locally with *Calendula lotion*, as per directions above.

A temporary inflammation with watering as the result of exposure to cold winds responds very nicely of *Aconite 30*. One dose will often clear up this condition.

If the trouble is due to dust bathe with *Euphrasia lotion* (ten drops of *Euphrasia Ø* to a wine glass of warm water) three or four times a day. Should the cat object to this lotion it may be further diluted and it will work just as well.

At times *Euphrasia* will clear up eye troubles better than *Calendula*, at others the reverse is the case.

If the eyelids stick together, smear a little *Calendula ointment* on them after treatment.

If the eyes are very mattery, bathe with *Saline* (a teaspoon of salt to a pint of water).

Cats which are out of condition often have the third eye partially over the eye and in such a case the general condition needs attention. Some kittens are born with their eyes open, or with inverted eyelids or eyelash troubles; these are congenital defects and a matter for a veterinary surgeon. Inverted eyelashes can be remedied by a slight operation. It would be inadvisable to use such stock for breeding.

Tuberculosis also affects cats' eyes but, of course, the disease would not be confined to the eyes.

Sometimes kittens get colds in their eyes which will water persistently for weeks on end. *Silica 6* two or three times a day for several weeks, followed by *Silica 30*, morning and evening, will sometimes clear up the trouble. In these cases wipe the eyes with cotton wool but do not use external applications of any kind.

FITS

Fits are not at all common in cats but kittens at teething time (4-6 months) are easily upset and sudden changes of food or environment at this time will sometimes induce convulsions. They may be the result of worms.

The symptoms are, the kitten may suddenly fall on its side, or it may cry and rush about, frothing at the mouth. It is temporarily quite unconscious and should be handled carefully or it may bite. It is better, if possible, and if it is not being very excitable or in a place where it cannot hurt itself or escape, to leave it where it is until it has quietened down and it can be confined to a quiet, dark room.

When the kitten has calmed down give *Chamomilla 6* every two hours for a few days, then stop and repeat if there is any recurrence of the trouble.

Feed on a light diet and keep quiet for some time, do not encourage it to play games lest it should get over excited.

FLEAS

Cats pick up fleas quite readily in the grass in summer, or from other infected animals, or from birds and mice which they may hunt and catch. Some kittens seem to attract these pests very easily.

Rub any good insect powder into the cat's coat but be sure that it has no *D.D.T.* in it as this is very poisonous to cats. If possible, powder the cat out of doors and leave the powder on for a few minutes, then let the cat shake itself and brush and comb it well. Be sure to powder the cat's sleeping quarters as well as the cat. Repeat the process every week or ten days until the coat is clean.

Internally, give one dose of *Sulphur 200* as this appears to discourage the pests. Repeat the dose once a week for three weeks. Fleas are also carriers of Tapeworm. Make sure the cat is free of this pest.

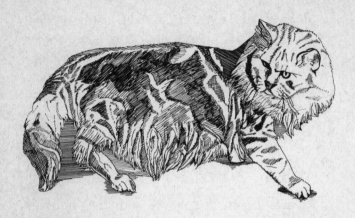

FRACTURES

In an accident where a cat may break a leg or get injured in a trap while hunting, this trouble must be attended to as soon as possible and if there is a break, set without delay by a veterinary surgeon. The administration of *Arnica Montana* 6 every two to four hours will help to overcome the shock and, later, *Symphytum 1x* given three times a day until the bone has united, will expedite the cure and keep the patient comfortable.

Some rickety kittens easily fracture their legs and *Silica* 6 at four hourly intervals for some time will strengthen the bones or, *Calcium Phos* 6 two or three times a day will benefit delicate kittens that do not actually show symptoms of rickets.

Silica 6 and *Calcium Phos* 6 can be given three hourly in alternation with good results where the kitten is delicate and bone development poor. The addition of *Bone Meal* to kittens' food is helpful to good bone formation.

HAIR BALL

As cats groom themselves with their tongues it is particularly necessary to comb them frequently to remove the shedded coat when they are moulting, particularly with long-haired cats. Short-haired cats, when coating profusely, also need this attention, otherwise the hair occasionally passes into the intestines and forms a hair ball. As a rule, cats enjoying their liberty eat grass and vomit up the hair which they have swallowed before it passes into the intestines. When they have not access to grass they may go off their food.

The cat should be dosed with *Liquid Paraffin* or *Olive Oil* in teaspoon doses once a week during the moulting season so as to avoid the formation of these hair balls. If a hair ball has formed give larger doses of the oil morning and evening until the cat passes or vomits the obstruction. An occasional dose of *Sulphur 30* will help at this time.

INDIGESTION

Cats occasionally suffer from indigestion, particularly those that may have been hand reared and possibly overfed.

The symptoms are occasional sickness and sometimes diarrhœa or constipation. The cat may eat well and later throw up all its food, or it may be temporarily off its food but not be very upset by these attacks.

Should the attack be caused by fat, rich food give *Pulsatilla 6* every three hours, this will help especially if the cat has diarrhœa with "no two motions alike."

In other cases *Carbo-Nux 6* after meals for a weak or two will generally tone up the digestive organs.

INFECTIOUS ENTERITIS

This is the most feared illness to which cats are prone; the death rate is enormous.

The disease is very infectious and more or less confined to kittens and cats under a year old. Quite often during an epidemic one kitten will show symptoms of catarrhal distemper and another of infectious enteritis. It is liable to appear after a spell of cold weather.

There is a period of latency when the kitten probably runs a temperature but, apart from lassitude, shows no other symptoms.

At the above mentioned stage, if it should be observed, *Aconite 30* night and morning for a day or two, might abort the condition. However, this stage is very seldom noticed and, in the next stage there is violent and persistent sickness and the little creature, during the course of the next few hours, wastes away to skin and bone. The temperature falls to subnormal, the kitten seeks water and may even try to lap some but it is as if it were afraid to do so; it sits over the bowl of water and, if it does lap it is again sick. It will lie about, only moving to be sick.

The vomiting often starts with an evacuation like the beaten white of an egg but it soon turns to bile. The kitten generally dies within 48 hours.

Give *Phosphorus 3* and *Bryonia Alb 3* in alternation every two hours and continue for 24 hours after all signs of sickness have disappeared. When the kitten has recovered give one dose of *Psorinum 200*.

It is essential to commence treatment on the first day, by the second it may be too far gone to react to any medicine.

JAUNDICE

This is not a common complaint in cats but it may occur as the result of a chill, apart from more serious causes such as organic diseases. It sometimes accompanies cat distemper.

The symptoms are loss of appetite, obstinate constipation and great depression; the cat wastes very quickly. The skin turns yellow (this is not easy to ascertain in cats but can be observed in the mouth and inside the ears in most cats). The urine is very highly coloured and scanty.

The treatment is *Chelidonium Major 6* two hourly in alternation with *Bryonia 6*.

The cat should be kept warm and it should have as much water as it will drink. Should it refuse all food it must be fed with small quantities of beef-tea or rabbit soup several times a day, or equal parts milk and soda water will sometimes be retained. All fats should be avoided.

After recovery *Sulphur 30* a dose morning and evening for two or three days will assist the cure.

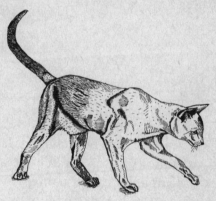

KIDNEY TROUBLES

Cats can get kidney trouble as the result of a chill and under these circumstances the treatment is as for Bladder trouble (see page 12).

In cases of Tuberculosis, the kidneys are also affected but in these cases it is far better to have the animal destroyed.

The symptoms of NEPHRITIS are, greater frequency in passing water, and there may be blood in the urine. There is marked thirst, the animal is depressed and listless, generally seeks warmth and it has an unthrifty appearance; the appetite may be retained.

In an acute attack, as the result of a chill, and if the condition is noticed very early, *Aconite 30* may relieve most of the symptoms. If, however, the condition appears to be chronic, which is not infrequently the case in old cats (and not very uncommon in young cats with a T.B. taint) it is better to have the animal put out of its misery.

Sometimes *Arsenicum Alb 30* will help; give one dose and do not repeat until the symptoms re-appear.

LICE

Cats pick up lice in hay or straw, in the grass or from other infected animals.

They are very small, whitish or greyish, looking life scurf, and they multiply at an amazing speed; they lay their eggs in the hair. The cat scratches incessantly.

The treatment is as for Fleas (see page 30).

If the cat is a great hunter or lives in the country and is liable to pick up lice it is as well to powder its coat at regular intervals as a preventative measure.

MANGE

This is fairly common in cats. It is one of the

few complaints which may be communicated to man.

The symptoms usually appear at first on the head, round the eyes and on the ears. The irritation is intense and worse for warmth. Owing to the irritation (which helps to distinguish this complaint from Ringworm) the cat gets very run down.

A cat affected with this trouble should be isolated and all its bedding, brushes and combs disinfected, or they may re-infect it.

For treatment bathe the cat once a week for three weeks in 2 ozs of Sulphurated Potash to 1 gallon of water. If there is more than one cat it is safer to bathe them all, as a protective measure, even if they do not show any symptoms of the complaint.

The toilet articles can be soaked in the same solution.

Keep the cat in the warm until it is quite dry and spray every place it has lain on with 40 per cent *Formaldehyde Solution*. Do not put the cat back into its quarters until the spray has dried and the fumes have evaporated.

Give one dose of *Sulphur 30* after each bath.

It will, of course, be necessary for persons to take precautions against the contagion to themselves, they should wash their hands with a suitable disinfectant and spray any of their garments on which the cat may have lain.

NEUTERING

Male cats which are kept as pets only should be neutered as an unneutered male, nearly, but not always, sprays and this is most unpleasant.

A whole male also strays, looking for mates, and gets himself involved in fights.

The operation, which should be performed by a qualified veterinary surgeon, is quite simple and it can be performed at any time after the age of three months. Before that age the testicles are not likely to have descended and the operation could not be performed. A cat can be neutered even after it has been used at stud and it settles down quite well as a household pet after it.

After the age of six months it is illegal to perform this operation without an anæsthetic.

It is advantageous to defer the operation until the cat has matured as the male head is attractive and this masculine appearance seldom develops if the neutering is carried out too early.

Very rarely is there any trouble after the operation but it is advisable to keep the cat quiet and warm for a few days and to administer a few doses of *Arnica Montana 6* to overcome any shock from the operation and to speed up the healing process.

Female cats are spayed, see under that heading.

OZOENA OR SNUFFLES—See Chronic Catarrh

PARALYSIS

When Paralysis is the result of an injury to the spine it is best to have the cat painlessly destroyed.

Cats sometimes get a temporary paralysis of the hind legs due to constipation.

It is advisable to change the diet. Milk acts as a mild aperient in many cats so this may be given freely, also give fish and, if the cat likes them, green vegetables with a little Olive Oil in them. Avoid meat with the exception of liver, which cats generally like and which tends to be laxative.

Give *Nux Vomica 3* three times a day as this will relieve the constipation and the pressure on the nerves, it will also tone up the digestion.

An enema might be necessary to clear the bowels.

A form of pseudo-paralysis from canker of the ear is not uncommon, for this see Canker (page 14).

PNEUMONIA

This may occur during the course of Distemper, especially if the initial rise of temperature is not noticed or, it may be the result of a chill.

The symptoms are rapid breathing, sometimes but not always a cough, and a sharp rise of temperature. The cat is off its food and disinclined to move; it may be thirsty.

Treatment in the intial stages is *Aconite 30* at hourly intervals for three doses only; this may abort the whole condition speedily.

If there is no improvement in 12 hours give *Bryonia 3* in alternation with *Phosphorus 3* every two hours.

Keep the cat warm, out of draughts but with plenty of fresh air and leave it alone as much as possible. Let it drink water which it probably will, or milk. Do not forcibly feed it for at least 48 hours.

Pneumonia responds very nicely to homoeopathic remedies which do not further lower the animal's resistance to the disease.

RHEUMATISM

Cats do not often suffer with Rheumatism but it does sometimes affect them.

A few doses of *Rhus Toxicodendron 30* in alternation with *Bryonia Alb 30* will generally give relief very quickly.

In one case which did not respond to the above mentioned remedies, the cat had been living out of doors in a damp place, and the suffering appeared to be localised in the hind-quarters. For days the cat moved as if it were crippled and unable to straighten the hind-quarters. On the assumption that this might be a case of which Dr. Burnett called "stored Gout", *Urtica Urens* Ø, five drops in 1 oz of hot water was given eight hourly. This cured the cat very quickly.

RICKETS

This is not a common complaint in cats but it does occur. It is a disease affecting kittens, the bones are soft, weak and bent. In bad cases the kitten walks on its ankles rather than on its toes. It moves with difficulty and has a generally unthrifty appearance with a dry stary coat. The animal is inclined to sit about instead of playing as a normal kitten should.

Kittens affected by Rickets are generally of unhealthy stock, though wrong feeding of the mother before birth may be partly responsible.

Diet is very important. Fresh Milk (Goat Milk is particularly good), Rabbit, Raw Meat, and Fish are essential and the kitten should be given two drops of *Haliverol* daily, and sprinkle a little bone meal on its food.

The kitten should be encouraged to move about and those in charge of it might induce this by playing with it. It should, of course, be housed in a dry warm place and exposed to sunlight as much as possible.

If the animal is undersized, cold, thin and looks helpless give *Silica 200*; one dose will give it grit and literally bring it to life. This can, if necessary, be repeated once a week for three weeks but one dose will often be all that is necessary.

Give *Calcium Phos 3x* in each meal.

The fat Scrofulous kitten that appears to be lazy rather than strikingly delicate needs a dose of *Calcium Carbonica 30* every two or three days over a period of two to three weeks.

If the mother cat is suspected of being responsible for the kitten's condition, she should be very carefully fed the next time she is pregnant, with Cod Liver Oil, Bone Meal and Yeast supplements.

The addition of the *five Phosphates* as supplied by Biochemic manufacturers (the publishers will give an address on receipt of a stamped addressed envelope), twice a day in her food will give her family a good start.

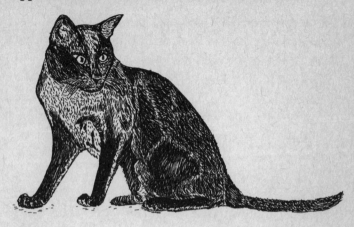

RINGWORM

This is another skin complaint which is not only very contagious from cat to cat and other animals but also to human beings.

Ringworm is due to a fungus and there are two varieties of the disease which affect the cat. The name is misleading as a cat does not always present the rings usually associated with the name.

The variety known as "Honeycomb Ringworm" can be distinguished by round-shaped scabs which appear with a central depression, usually on the head, ears or paws.

The other type generally starts on the same places but, if unchecked, it may spread to all parts of the cat.

The lesions are small, dry, grey and scaly-looking at first. They spread if neglected or overlooked; the hair breaks off and quite large rings form. There is little irritation.

The great difficulty with this disease is that cats can be carriers of the complaint without themselves showing any sign of it. Under these circumstances, should the cat be immune from the contagion, its presence will not be suspected until the cat has kittens which, in a few weeks, develop the lesions.

Treatment is as for Mange (see page 37).

In view of the fact that a cat can act as a carrier in case there is an outbreak it is essential in a Cattery to wash every animal in the place.

Three baths at weekly intervals generally suffice to clear the condition completely unless the Cattery and everything with which the cat may have been in contact has not been disinfected with 40 per cent *Formaldehyde* spray, or fumigated.

In bathing the animal the solution must reach every part but care must be taken to prevent any getting into the eyes.

The coat must not be rinsed but well dried and the cat kept in a warm room until the coat is perfectly dry. Give the animal a warm drink or meal before returning it to its isolation quarters where it must be confined for three weeks.

The isolation quarters can be sprayed while

the cat is being bathed and dried but be sure that the fumes have evaporated and the spray has dried before returning the cat to these quarters. It is advisable to cover the mouth and nose with a handkerchief while spraying as the solution is very strong.

Give one dose of *Sulphur* 200 after each bath.

SCURF or DANDRUFF

This is a form of Eczema, the cat has a dry skin and the dandruff or scurf is sometimes profuse.

The animal is out of condition. Regular grooming will help and a change of diet is also of assistance. The trouble may be due to worms.

As the skin scales with ringworm it is advisable to make sure that the trouble is mere debility and not incipient skin trouble.

Sulphur 6 given morning and evening for a few weeks will improve the animals general condition.

Natrum Muriaticum 6, to be given in the same manner if worms are suspected as the cause.

SPAYING

This is the removal of the ovaries in a female cat. It can, as in neutering males, be performed at any age. It is commonly done these days when a female is wanted only as a pet. It has also to be performed when, for any reason, a queen may have difficulty in giving birth to her kittens.

The operation is a major one and the cat should be kept warm, quiet and carefully watched for about a week after her return home, she then has to have the stitches removed.

Give *Arnica 6* two or three times a day beginning the day before the cat is to have the operation and for a few days after it.

A little *Calendula Lotion* (10 drops of Ø to a wine glass of water) may be dabbed on the scar to promote rapid healing.

TEETH and TEETHING

Kittens start their first set of teeth very early and the milk teeth are complete within a few weeks. There are fourteen in the top jaw and twelve in the lower.

The second teething begins at about four months and the permanent teeth, thirty in number, are generally all through by 6 to 7 months of age.

At this time the kitten should be protected from possible infections and contagions. It should be fed suitably and sometimes a large meaty bone helps when the kitten is changing its teeth.

A healthy kitten usually gets through teething without any trouble but it is, nevertheless, a trying time and it is, therefore, more easily upset both mentally and physically than at other times. Some delicate kittens get very run down during these months.

Any abrupt change of environment or diet at this time may cause convulsions but these cease when the permanent teeth are through (see under Fits, page 29).

Calcium Phos 6 given two or three times a day helps kittens through the teething period.

Older cats form tartar on their teeth and this should be scraped off periodically by a Veterinary Surgeon. The cat's breath becomes foul and an excess of tartar will cause inflammation of the gums; if this is very bad the cat will dribble and have difficulty in eating. The teeth also get loose and decayed. All loose teeth should be extracted.

Abscesses on the face are often due to bad teeth and, at times, in old cats the eye teeth get over long and they can be shortened by a Veterinary Surgeon if they cause trouble.

After scaling, swab the mouth with *Calendula Lotion* (a teaspoon of the Ø to half a cup of water).

TUBERCULOSIS

This disease is very contagious from one cat to another and it would be very unwise to risk an infected cat running around anywhere near children.

Once a case is definitely established, the cat is obviously ill, losing flesh, with chronic diarrhœa, a cough or a continued rise of temperature. The temperature may vary but a persistent reading of 102° or over is very ominous.

The disease can attack almost any organ and the eyes are frequently affected.

In a fully developed case it is better to have the animal destroyed immediately.

It is likely that many cats which are unthrifty have a T.B. taint. In such cases, if the disease has not developed, a course of *Bacillinum 30*, a dose once a week for a few weeks may well arrest it and bring about a reaction leading to an improvement in every way.

Meat unfit for human consumption should never be fed to cats raw. It seems that birds are now very subject to the Avian type of T.B. and these, too, can be a source of contagion to cats.

TUMOURS

These are sometimes found in old cats and they may be either benign or malignant. A veterinary examination will determine the variety. The former causes little discomfort but the latter may, at a late stage, cause great pain with a discharge of blood-stained pus and there is, generally, a rapid wasting away. Tumours may develop in any part of the body.

Where there is a malignant growth and the animal is in pain it is much kinder to have the cat painlessly destroyed.

Benign tumours of the mammary glands of queens often respond very nicely to the administration of *Phytolacca 30*, morning and evening for a few days.

It is fairly simple to distinguish between an abscess and a tumour. The former, though it may be hard when first noticed is painful to the touch, its appearance is sudden and development rapid, whereas with a tumour the development is slow. Further, an abscess in a cat is generally accompanied by a rise of temperature.

VOMITING

Simple vomiting may be due to a cat's propensity for eating grass in order to get rid of anything, such as hair, which has upset its digestion and it may be disregarded.

Some cats are frequently sick with no other symptoms of indisposition. If this continues give *Ipecacuanha* 6, a few doses three times a day will soon give relief.

It is easy to distinguish between simple vomiting and Infectious Enteritis or the kind sometimes seen in one of the cat Influenzas in which the cat is rapidly prostrated.

Simple sickness is generally due to a digestive disturbance and when the attack is over treat as for Indigestion (see page 33).

Cats subject to liver troubles and gastric complaints sometimes suffer, particularly at changes of weather; they vomit and show mild catarrhal symptoms, lethargy or no inclination to move at all, there is no thirst and seldom any temperature. A few doses of *Chelidonium Majus* 3 at three hourly intervals helps very quickly.

The cat should be protected from violent changes of temperature and kept in the warm until the symptoms pass.

Where the symptoms are worse during damp weather give *Natrum Sulph. 30* one a day for a few doses.

WORMS

Most kittens and cats get worms occasionally and they may get rid of them or have them without causing any apparent harm.

They are subject to two kinds of worms, the round worm and the tapeworm.

The usual symptoms are irregular appetite, sometimes they are voracious and at other times they refuse food; the coat is "Starey" and the cat remains thin. Sometimes the haw of the eye showing may indicate the presence of worms.

Cats often vomit round worms.

For round worms give *Chenopodium ∅* in pilule form night and morning for a few weeks and later one dose of *Cina 200* which can be repeated in a week.

For Tape worms give *Filix Mas. 3x* night and morning for a few weeks and at the end of the period one dose of *Filix Mas. 200*.

In obstinate cases of Tape Worms, especially if accompanied by slimy, bloody motions, give *Mercurius Corrosivus 6* morning and evening for a week or until the symptoms are alleviated.

Natrum Phos 6x, morning and evening, for weeks at a time corrects the acid condition conducive to worms.

WOUNDS

Cats living natural lives, as they all should, often get themselves injured in one way or another.

In cases of serious street accidents (such as being hit by a car), a Veterinary Surgeon should examine the cat as soon as possible as the injury may be far more serious than is apparent, but while awaiting this examination give the cat *Arnica Montana 6* every hour for

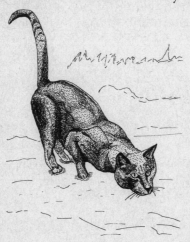

four or more doses after which lengthen the period between doses; this will help to allay the shock.

Calendula Lotion (one teaspoonful of the Ø to half a cup of water) is a first class dressing for all wounds, it inhibits the growth of micro-organisms.

For punctured wounds such as bites and those made by sharp-pointed instruments or splinters give *Ledum 6* internally every two hours in the place of *Arnica* and externally apply *Calendula Lotion* (10 drops of the Ø in a wine glass of water). *Hypericum Lotion* (10 drops of the Ø to a wine glass of water) is also excellent as an external remedy.

For injured nerves, lacerations and crushed parts etc., where the pain is very great apply *Hypericum Lotion* (10 drops in a wine glass of water) externally and give *Hypericum 6* internally every two hours.

In bad cases do not remove the dressing more than once in 24 hours but moisten it with the lotion when it becomes dry.

GENERAL HINTS

Cats enjoy a varied diet. They have their own

preferences in the matter of food, some like milk, others do not. Some like fish others prefer meat.

It is always wise, when purchasing a cat or kitten to learn exactly how it has been fed and to avoid making any sudden change in its diet. Cats are nervous creatures and the change of environment and people is sufficient for them to cope with during the first few days.

An adult cat requires two meals a day, morning and evening. The morning feed may consist of raw oat flakes soaked in hot milk and given to the cat when cool, or porridge and milk or any of the breakfast cereals may be acceptable. The cat will soon show its preference. The second meal should consist of rabbit, fish or meat and vegetables. Some cats like tinned cat foods such as "Kit-E-Kat'" as a change. Meat "unfit for human consumption" should always be well cooked.

Meals should be given at regular times.

Kittens need feeding more frequently. Farex with milk makes a good start to the day or Quaker or Scotts' Oats raw, soaked in hot milk and fed when cool. Meat or fish cut small for dinner. A drink of milk (Goats' milk is the best possible for kittens) for tea and more meat or fish with well-cooked vegetables mixed in for supper. Lightly boiled eggs, milk puddings or grated cheese are acceptable changes. The amount will have to be increased gradually to allow for growth.

Fresh, clean water should be available at all times.

HOUSE TRAINING

A new arrival or any sick cat which is confined to the house must be given a sanitary tray. As a rule cats are clean creatures. A good queen will teach her kittens house manners and the use of the tray. A deep tray may suit an adult cat but kittens need shallow trays for ease of getting in and out. Anything absorbent may be used in the tray; ashes or peat moss are probably the nicest for the purpose; some people use. paper or dried earth. The tray must be kept in the same place at all times and the cat shown where it is; if it is moved the cat may soil the original place. Trays must be cleaned regularly as no self respecting cat will use a dirty one. Enamel baking tins are very suitable as they are easy to keep clean. If a disinfectant is used, *T.C.P.*, or a *Pine disinfectant* is pleasant and safe.

GROOMING

All cats should be regularly groomed. Young kittens which are groomed regularly soon get used to it and often enjoy it. Some cats are difficult to groom and in these cases it is better to do a bit at a time and cease if the animal is getting too upset. Long-haired cats need more attention than short-haired but both types need regular grooming.

Stiff bristled brushes help to remove a lot of hair. Short-haired cats may be combed with a fairly fine comb to remove any loose hairs and then well rubbed down with the bare hands or a silk handkerchief, this will give a good gloss and the cat will enjoy it as it will be regarded as petting.

Eyes and ears should be attended to at the same time and small kittens should be watched under the tail as they sometimes have accidents in their furry trousers.

EYES

Kittens open their eyes about the tenth day after birth. As a rule they give no trouble but occasionally they stick and are troublesome. This should not be neglected; if they look healthy but stick only at night smear a little *Calendula Ointment* along the lids, this may be all that is necessary. If, however, they get worse and discharge matter bathe with *Saline* (one teaspoon of salt to one pint of water) and then smear with *Calendula Ointment*. Give, internally, one dose of *Pulsatilla 30* every second or third day. If the remedy is in pilule form, crush one and place it under the tongue of a tiny kitten.

GRASS

Cats having liberty are fond of grass, which acts as an emetic and long-haired cats seem to use it mainly for that purpose as an aid in getting rid of hairs that they have swallowed. If a cat is confined in a flat, grass may be grown in boxes for it.

OUT OF CONDITION

Sometimes, for no apparent reason cats get thin and fussy with their food or the appetite may be increased. These symptoms are sometimes accompanied by loose, yellow stools and abdominal distension. Five drops of *Alfalfa* Ø is an excellent tonic, given in food two or three times a day for a few weeks.

TEMPERATURE

The normal temperature of a cat is 101.4. It is best to take it in the rectum though cats frequently object to this. It can be taken under the arm or leg but one needs to be sure that it is accurately taken there as the thermometer is liable to slip, therefore, it is advisable to assume the temperature to be about one degree more than the actual reading when it is taken under the arm or leg. In most animals it is wise to take the temperature after it has been quiet for some time as excitement of any kind will sometimes cause a rise in temperature. Any reading over 102° should be carefully watched.

FOODS FOR INVALIDS

If invalid cats will eat anything during sickness it is of great help. Water should be available at all times, as they may take this voluntarily in preference to anything else.

Slippery Elm Food is very good. Beaten up egg with a few drops of brandy or whisky is good in great weakness. So is Brand's Essence.

Sometimes a cat will eat raw meat, fish or rabbit, or even custard may be appreciated and a sick animal may take sufficient to keep it going.

It is not necessary to recourse to forcible feeding for 48 hours but if food is refused after this period a small quantity should be given about every two hours. Feeding liquid food through a hypodermic syringe *with the needle removed* is very easy and provided a cloth is put round the cat's neck to prevent the food getting onto the cat itself, this method of feeding need disturb the animal very little.

Provided that there are no gastric symptoms and the temperature is not very high, raw meat cut up small, pushed down the throat morning and evening will keep the animal going until it starts to eat of its own accord.

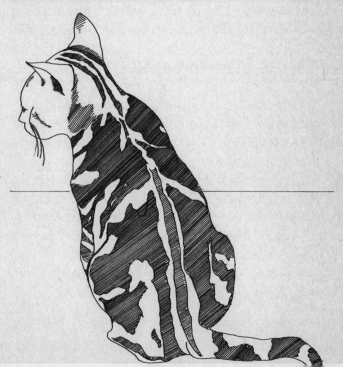

GIVING MEDICINES

As homoeopathic pilules are small and pleasant to take they are easier to administer to cats than other medicines.

Open the cat's mouth and drop the pill down the throat and close the mouth quickly. Watch carefully to be sure that it has been swallowed; some cats are very skilful at ejecting pills after they appear to have been swallowed and they may later be discovered in their beds.

If a cat is particularly difficult (and some are), the pilules may be crushed and placed up the side of the mouth or dissolved in water and given in this way or, if the animal is eating, the medicine can be given in the food.

POTENCIES

In acute conditions the remedies must be given more frequently until the cat gets relief. When there are signs that the symptoms are relieved or there is improvement, i.e., when the vomiting or diarrhœa stops (if that is the trouble), or the cat seems easier and appears to be sleeping, or assumes an easier attitude it is a sign that the medicine is doing its work and WHILE IMPROVEMENT CONTINUES THERE IS NO NEED TO REPEAT THE DOSE. If the prescriber is not sure that the remedy selected is the correct one it is advisable to keep to the lower potencies up to the sixth (3x, 3, 4x, 4, 5x, 5, 6x and 6). The potency is denoted by the figure after the name of the remedy.

The low potencies work just as well but not so quickly as the higher potencies which work rapidly and deeply if correctly prescribed, but which may, if incorrectly used, cause complications.

In acute diseases it is well to continue the medicine for 24 to 48 hours, at increasing intervals, after the animal appears to be cured.

Note the sign Ø means mother tincture and remedies marked in this are in liquid form.

The author of this book has had special condition tablets (also in powder form) made for cats and these are recommended, they are known as *SHEPPARD HOMOEOPATHIC CONDITION REMEDY* supplied by Ransley-Robinson Research Laboratories Ltd., 3b Manor Parade, Durrington, Sussex.

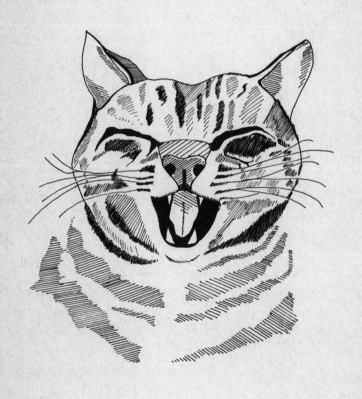